Daddy's got Dementia

Written by Emma Anius
Illustrated by Tamina White

A note to the reader

If a loved one has recently been diagnosed with dementia, or you have been on this journey for some time, firstly I would like to say I am sorry- I feel your pain, and you are not alone. It will be challenging, but to go down the road of caring for someone you love, is a road worth traveling.

'Daddy's got Dementia' was written to help you capture and hold onto those precious moments that often get overlooked.   You will be able to look back at the times you spent with your loved one and smile, knowing that the small moments are the ones that truly meant the most. The memories you capture with this book will be ones you can cherish and hold onto forever knowing that they will never be forgotten.

The journey you are about to embark on, will be like no other, and I hope we can help you get through the roller coaster ride that is looking after a loved one that has been diagnosed with dementia. To hopefully allow you to see the brighter side to the harder moments in life, giving you comfort in knowing that you are not alone on this journey.

There will be good times, there will be hard times, but if there is one piece of advice that I would like to share, it would be to know that no matter how hard things may seem, no matter what happens, everything is going to be OK.

Daddy's got dementia
But it's OK
He still likes to laugh run and play

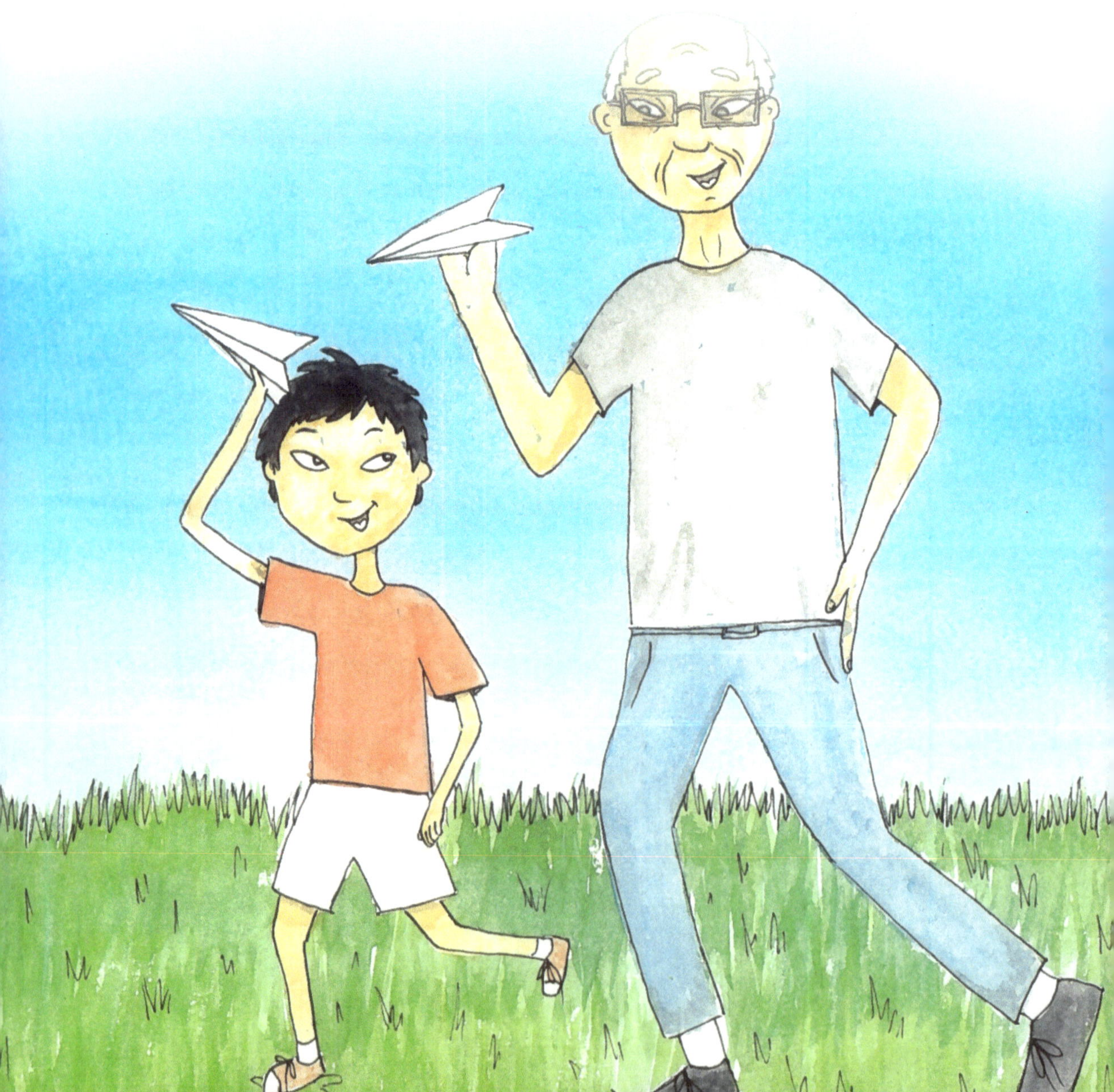

What are your top 3 favorite things that you love to do with your daddy?

Daddy's got dementia
But it's OK
He still likes to cook, read books,
and pray

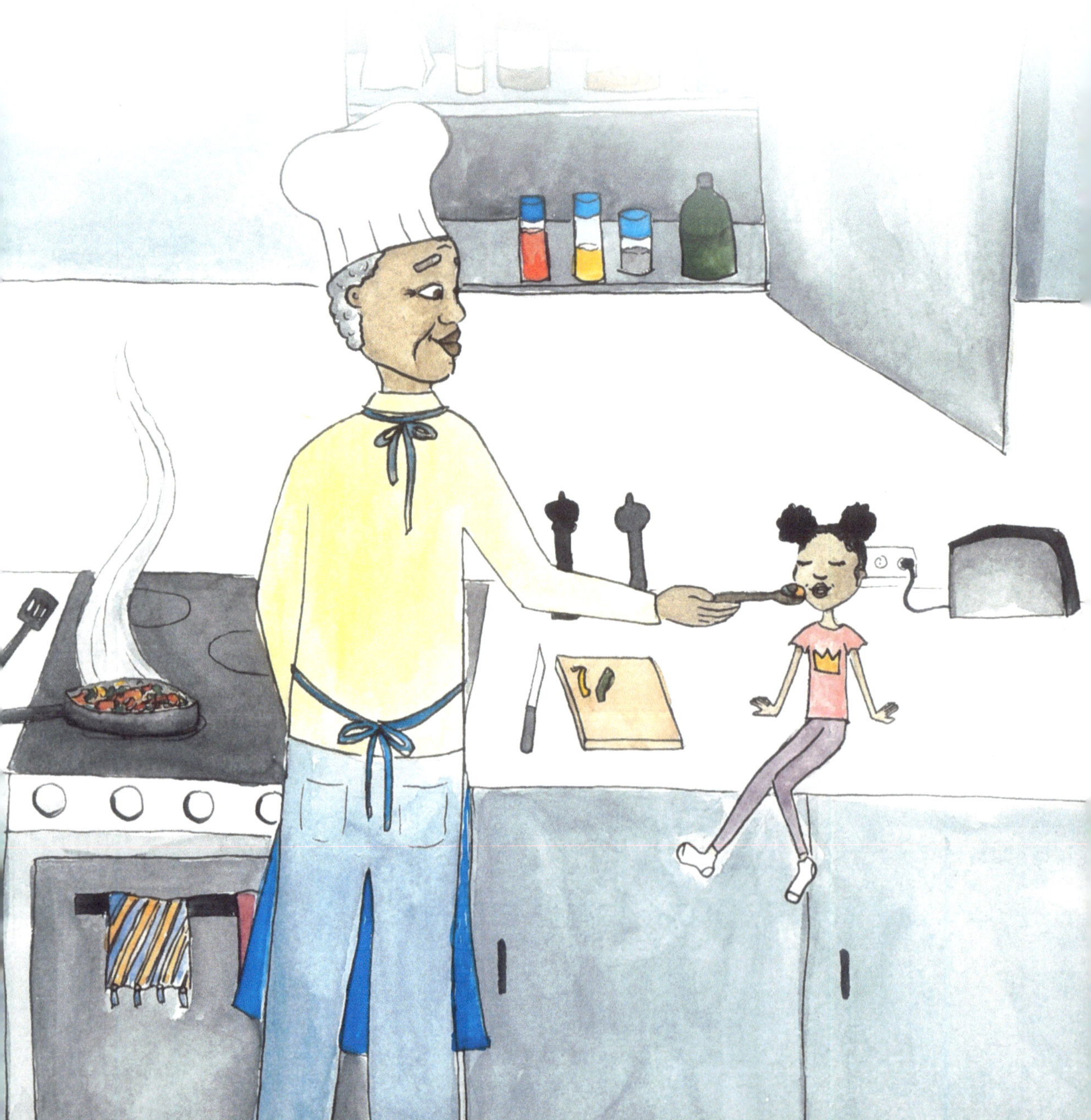

What is your daddy's favorite recipe?

INGREDIENTS:

DIRECTIONS:

Notes

Daddy's got **dementia**
But it's **OK**
He still likes to have **brunch** at his favorite **cafe**

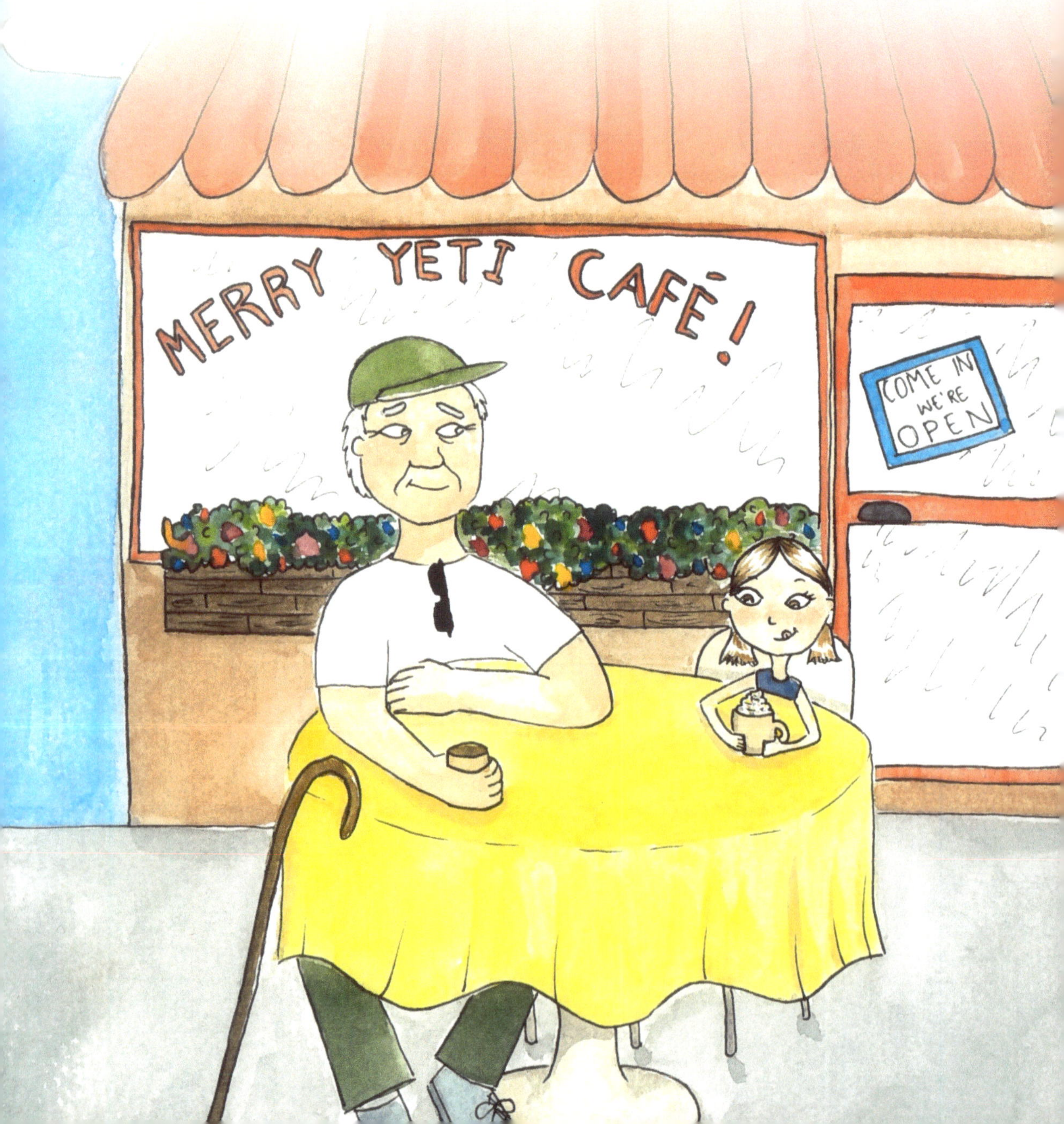

Place a picture of you and daddy
at his favorite cafe.

Place picture here

Do you have any happy memories about
going out to eat with your daddy?

Daddy's got dementia
But it's OK,
He comes to cheer at my ballet

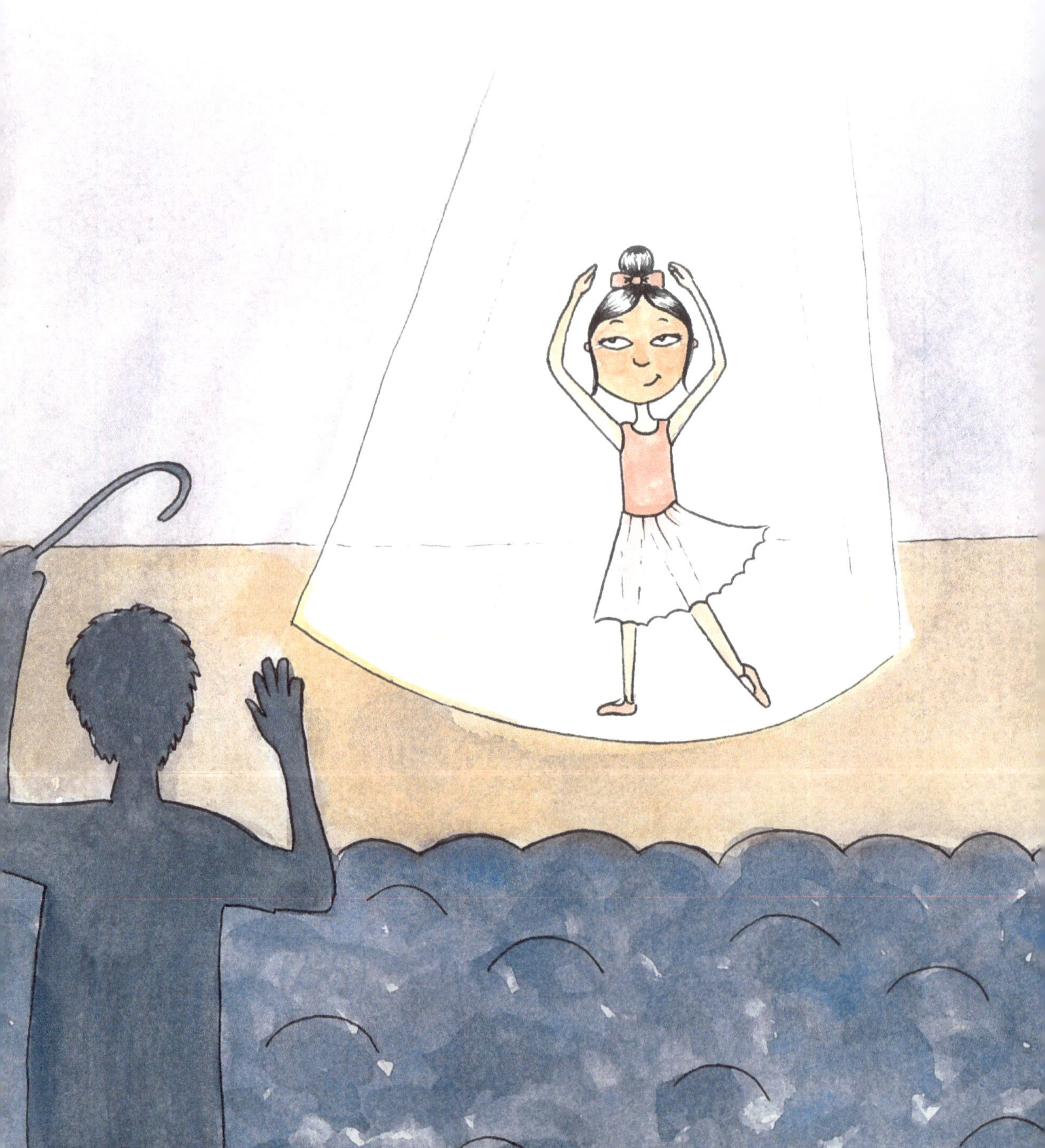

What is daddy's favorite sports team or sport to watch?

____

____

____

Do you have any stories you want to share about your daddy?

____

____

____

____

____

____

____

____

____

Daddy's got dementia
But it's OK
He still likes to buy mom a
bouquet on Valentine's Day.

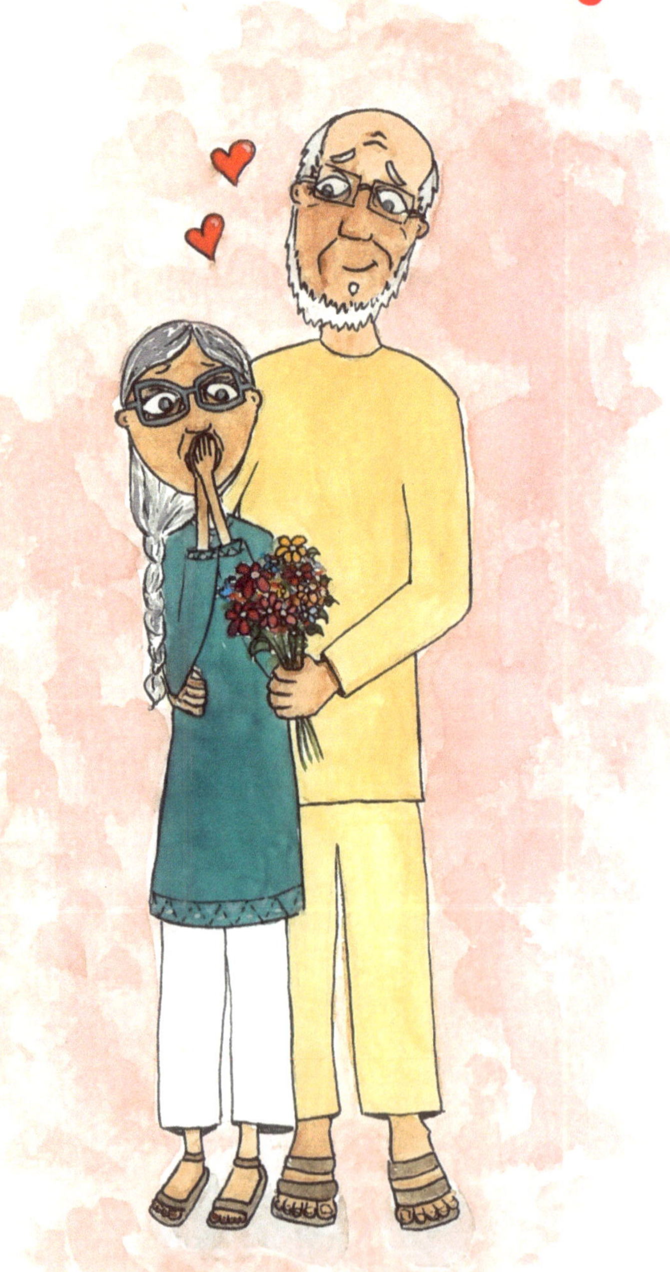

Write down a happy memory you have with your daddy.

Daddy's got **dementia**
But it's **OK**
We get to paint together and put
our art on **display**

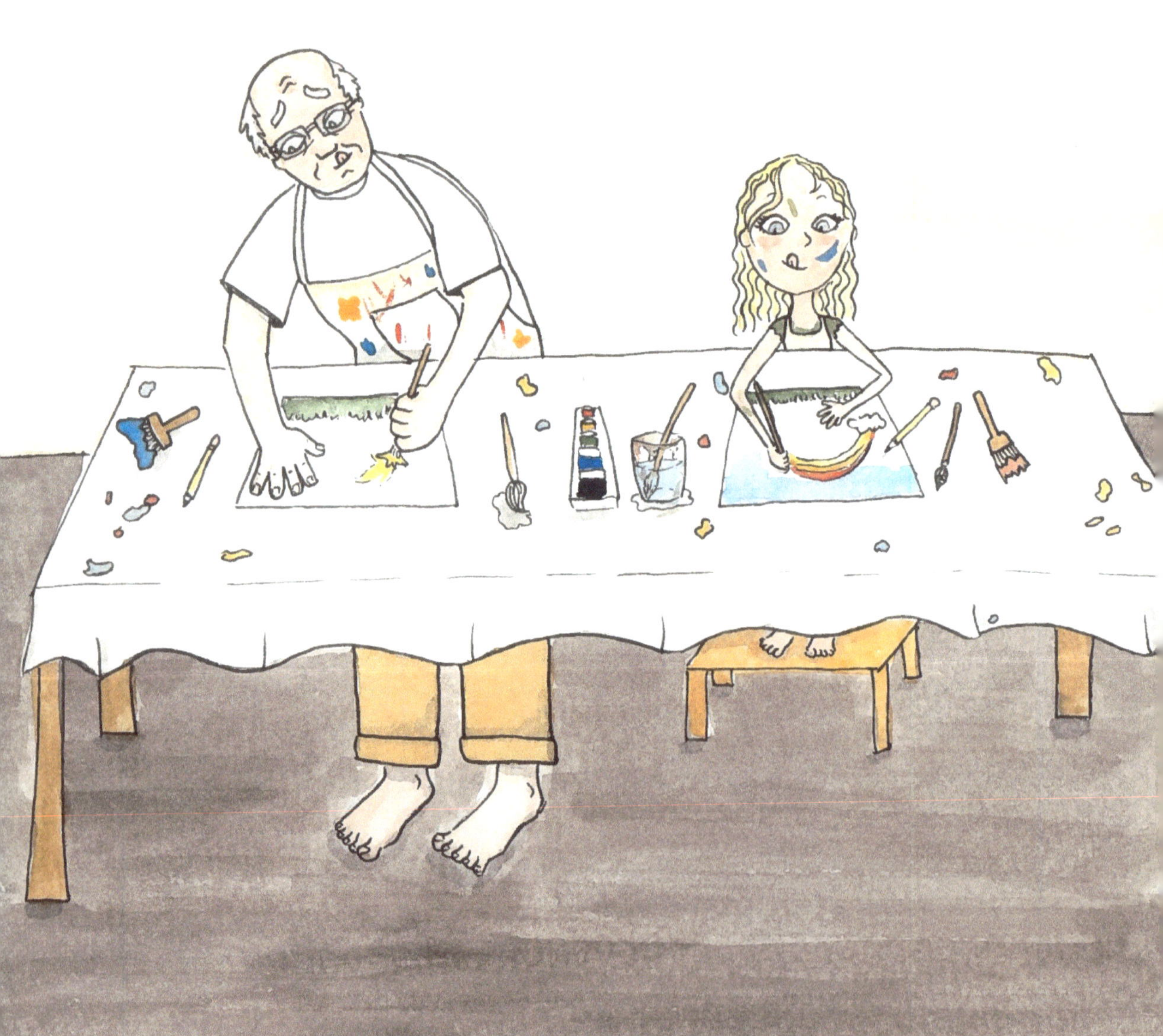

What do you and your daddy like doing together?

____

____

____

____

____

____

____

Place picture here

Daddy's got dementia
But it's OK
We still whistle our favorite song
"Sittin' On The Dock of the Bay"

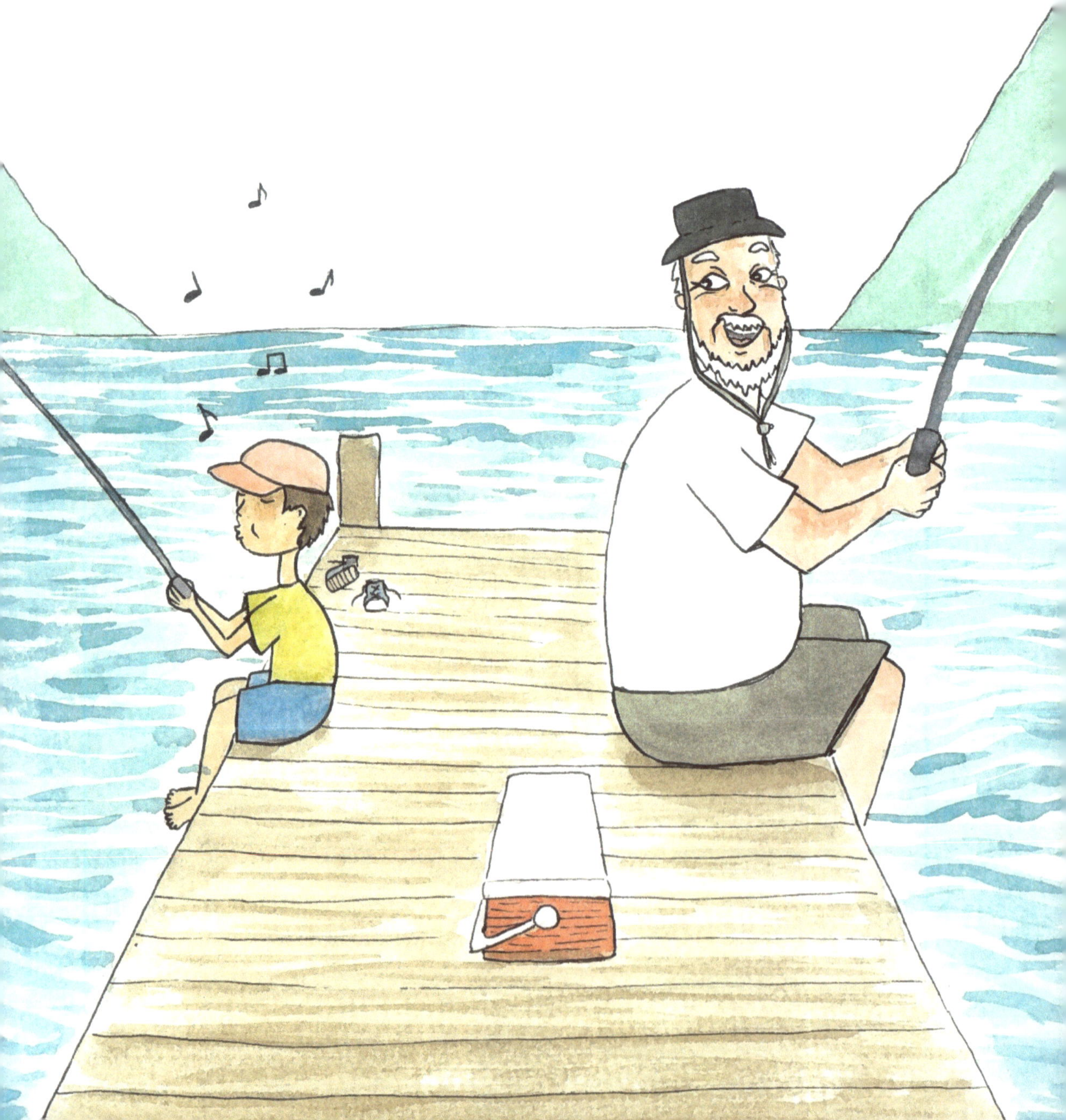

What is daddy's favorite
song to sing with you?

____

____

____

Do you have any sweet memories to share?

____

____

____

____

____

____

____

____

____

Daddy's got dementia
But it's OK
He lets me brush his hair, even
though it's gray

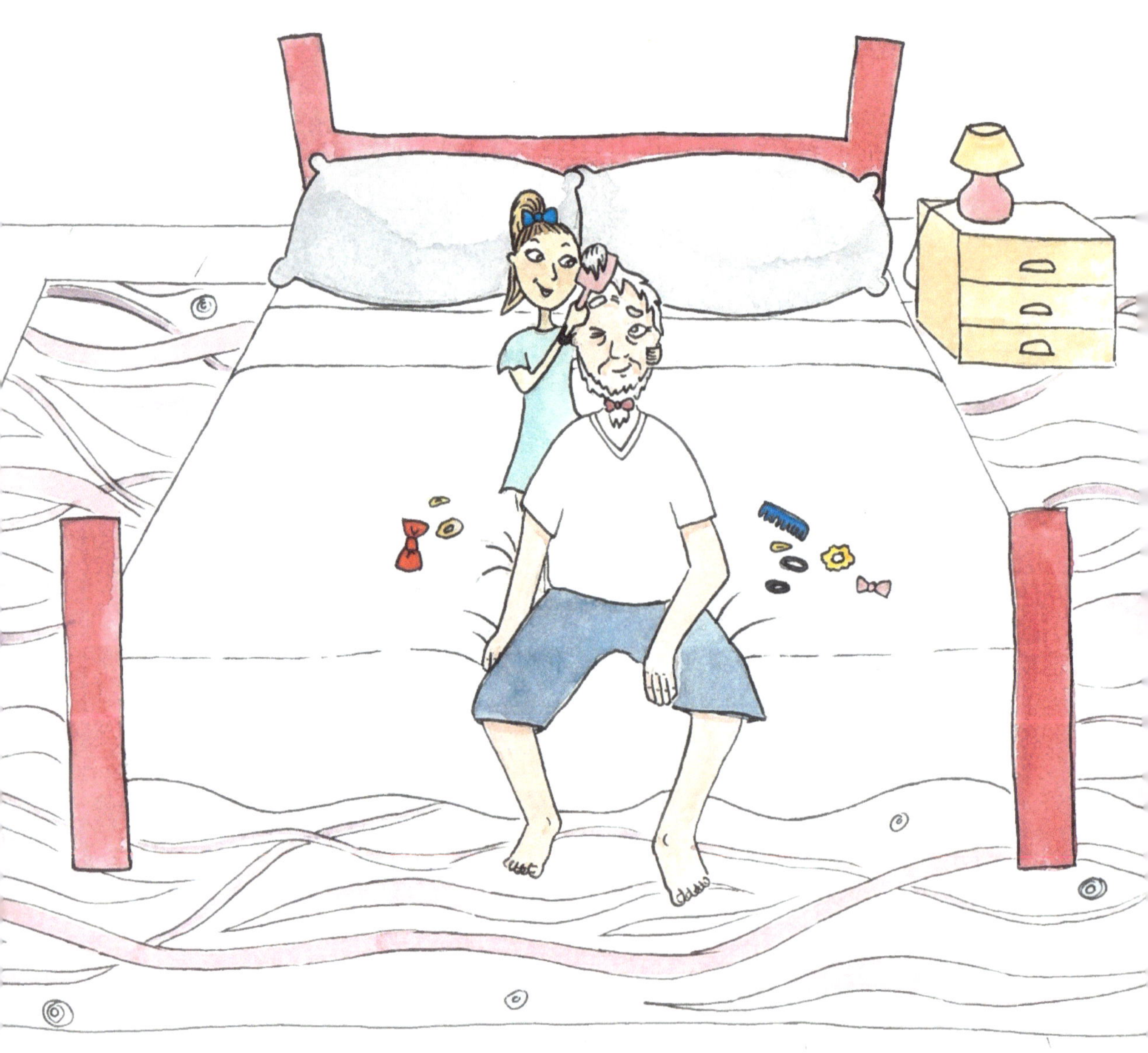

Share a lovely picture that you have with your daddy all dressed up.

What is this picture about?

____

____

____

____

____

Place picture here

Place picture here

What is this picture about?

____

____

____

____

____

____

Daddy's got dementia
But it's OK
Even though sometimes he tries
to run away

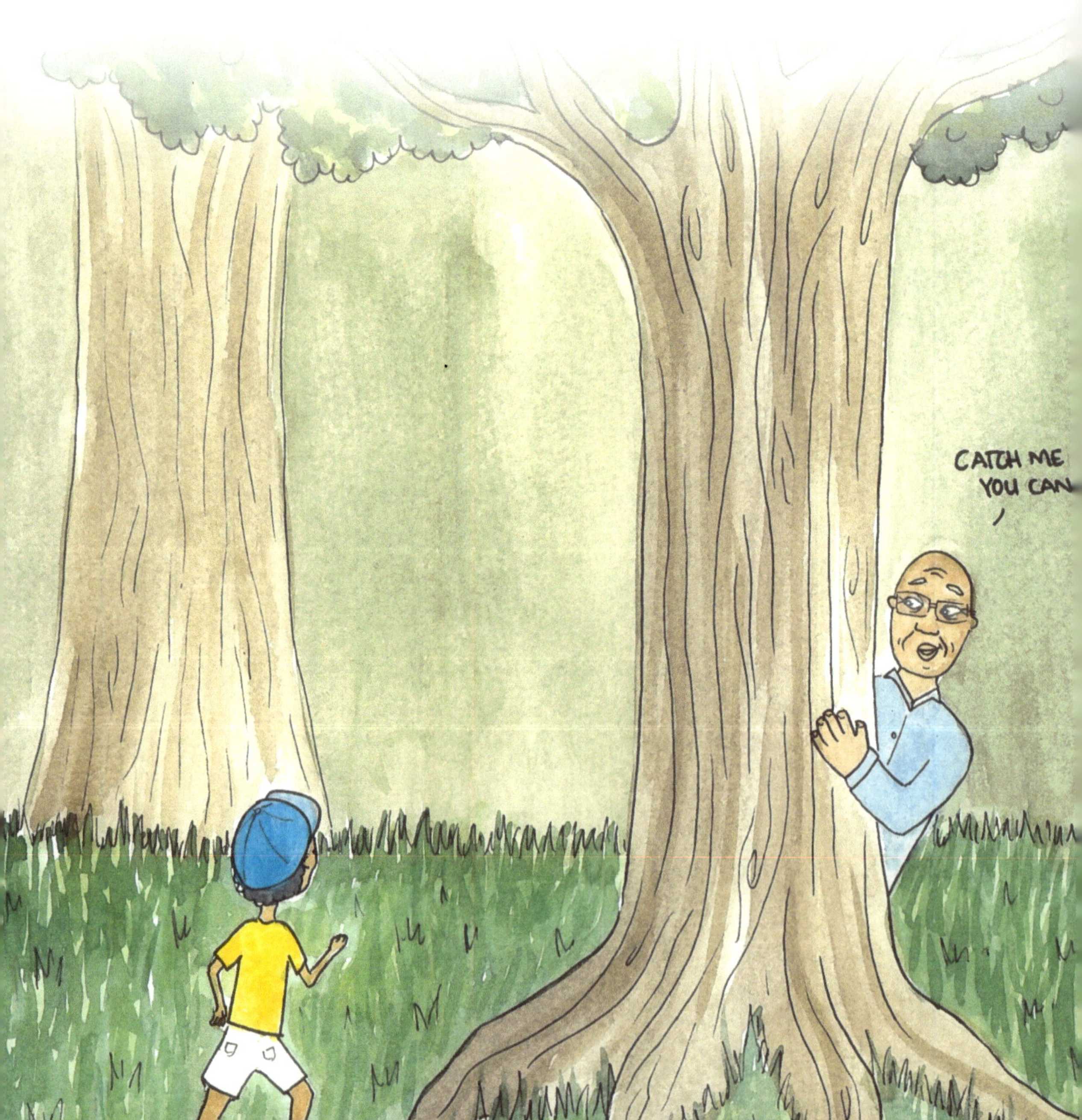

Do you have any memories of your dad trying to run away?

Daddy's got dementia
But it's OK
He sometimes forgets- he thought it was February but it's really May

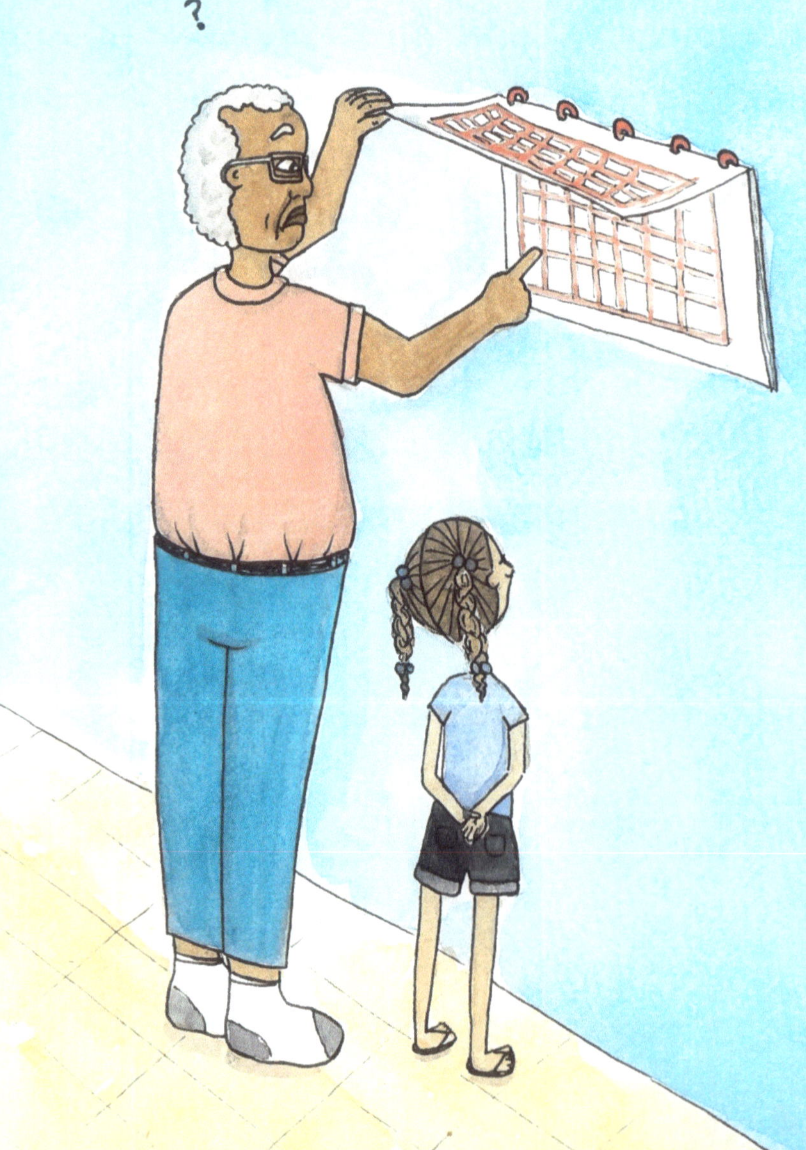

What is your favorite memory with your daddy?

Daddy's got dementia
But it's OK
He tells us the same story, but
we are happy to listen all day

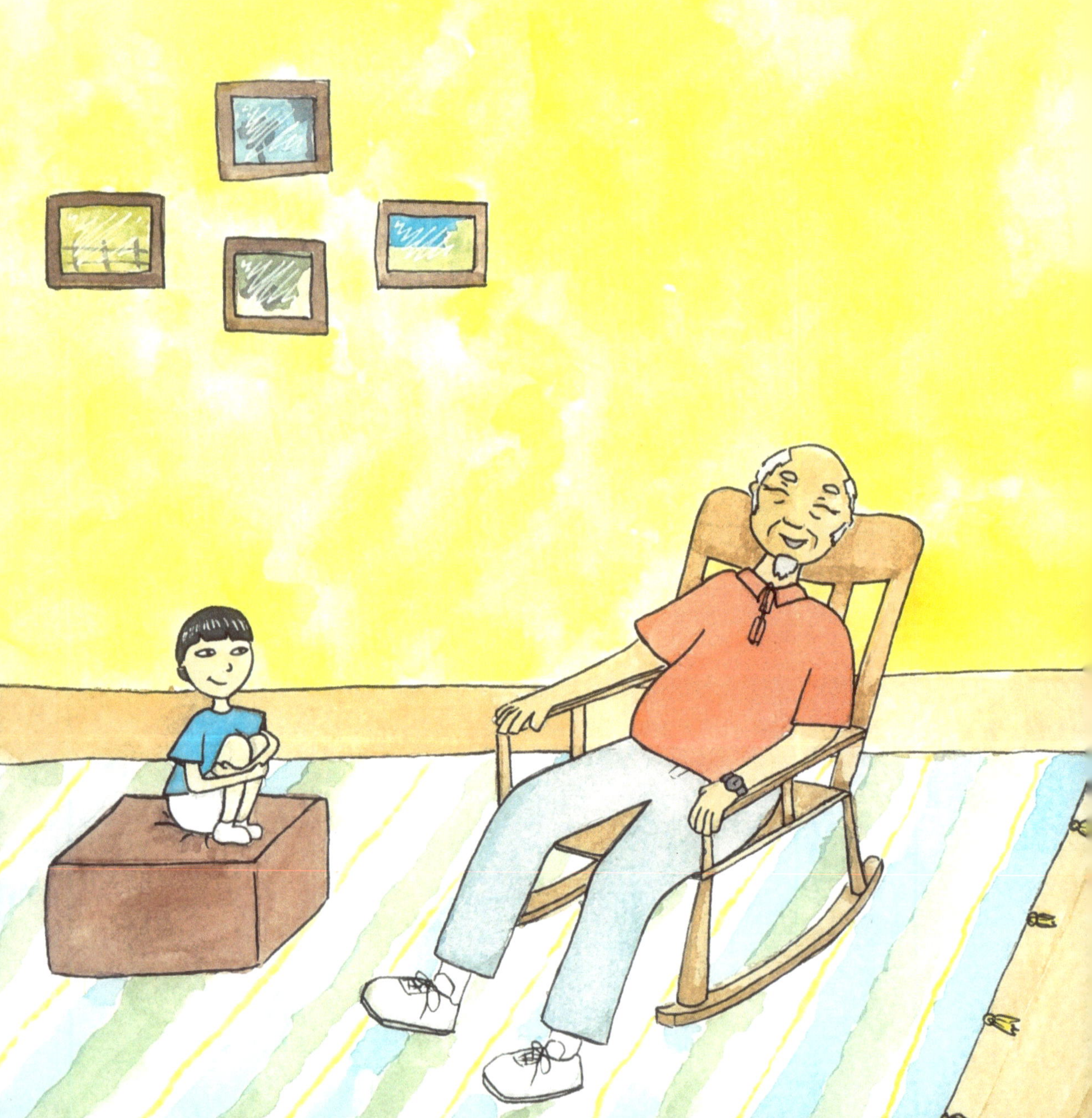

What is daddy's favorite story
that he loves to tell?

Daddy's got dementia
But it's OK
I thought he forgot, but he remembered my birthday!

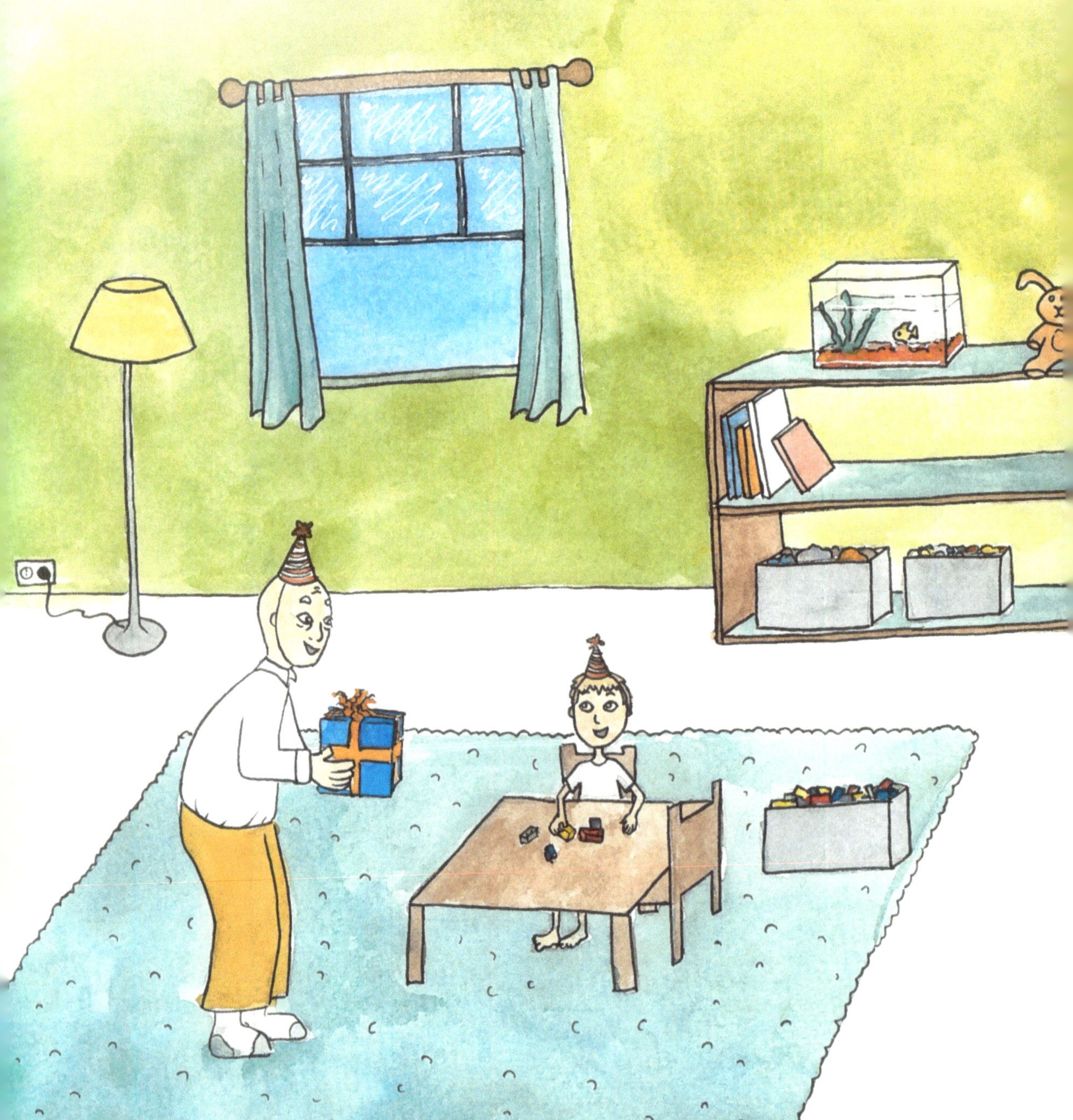

Do you have a happy birthday memory with your daddy?

____

____

____

____

____

Place a picture with you and daddy on your birthday

____

____

Daddy's got dementia
But it's OK
We are here to love him all the
way

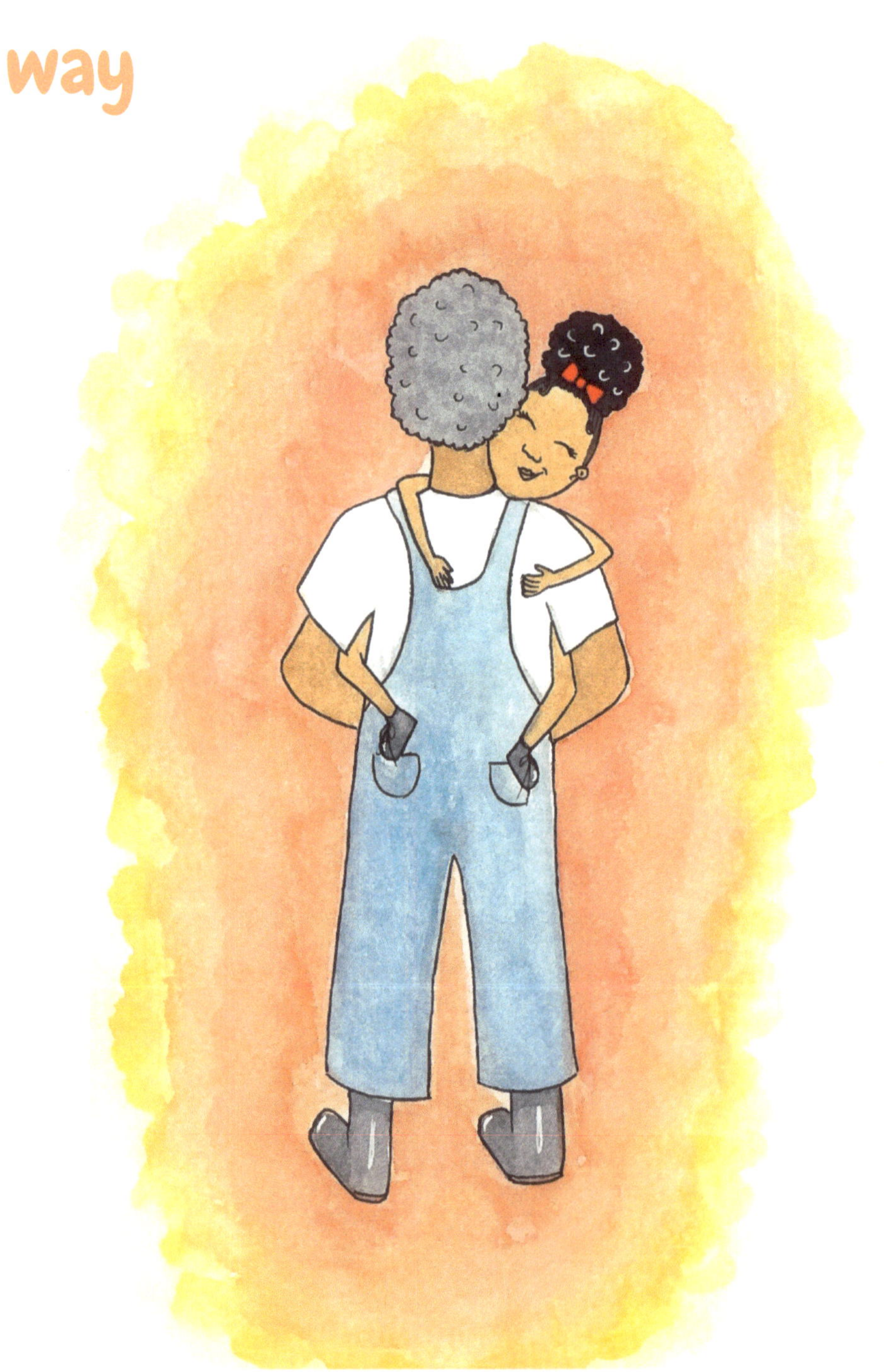

Write down some of the favorite things you love about your daddy.

Daddy's got dementia
But it's OK
I know he loves me, even if he
cannot say

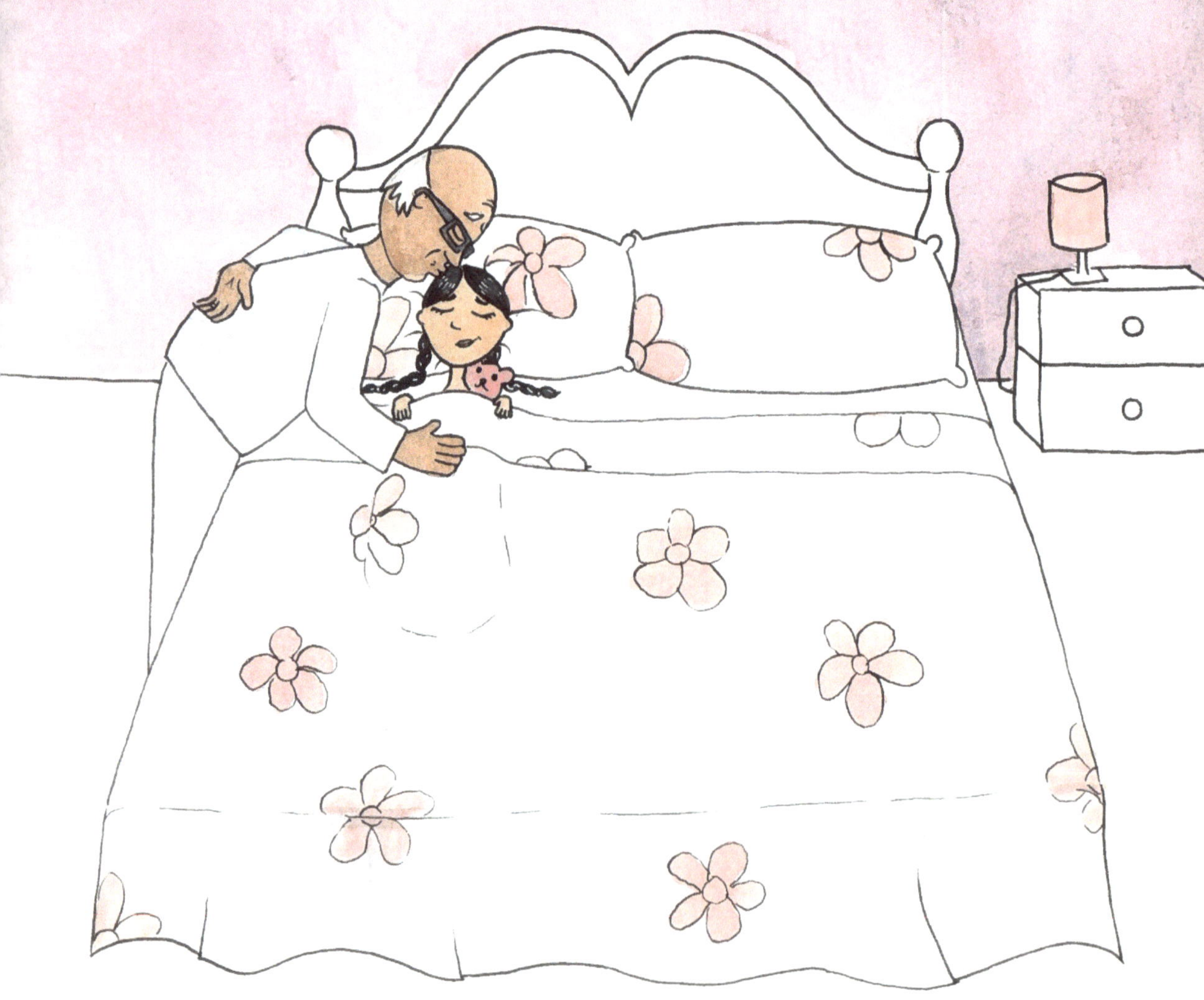

Do you have a sweet memory you want to share about your daddy?

____

____

____

____

____

____

____

____

Place a happy picture of you and daddy here

Daddy's got dementia
But it's OK
Sometimes he gets a little mad,
but we love him anyway

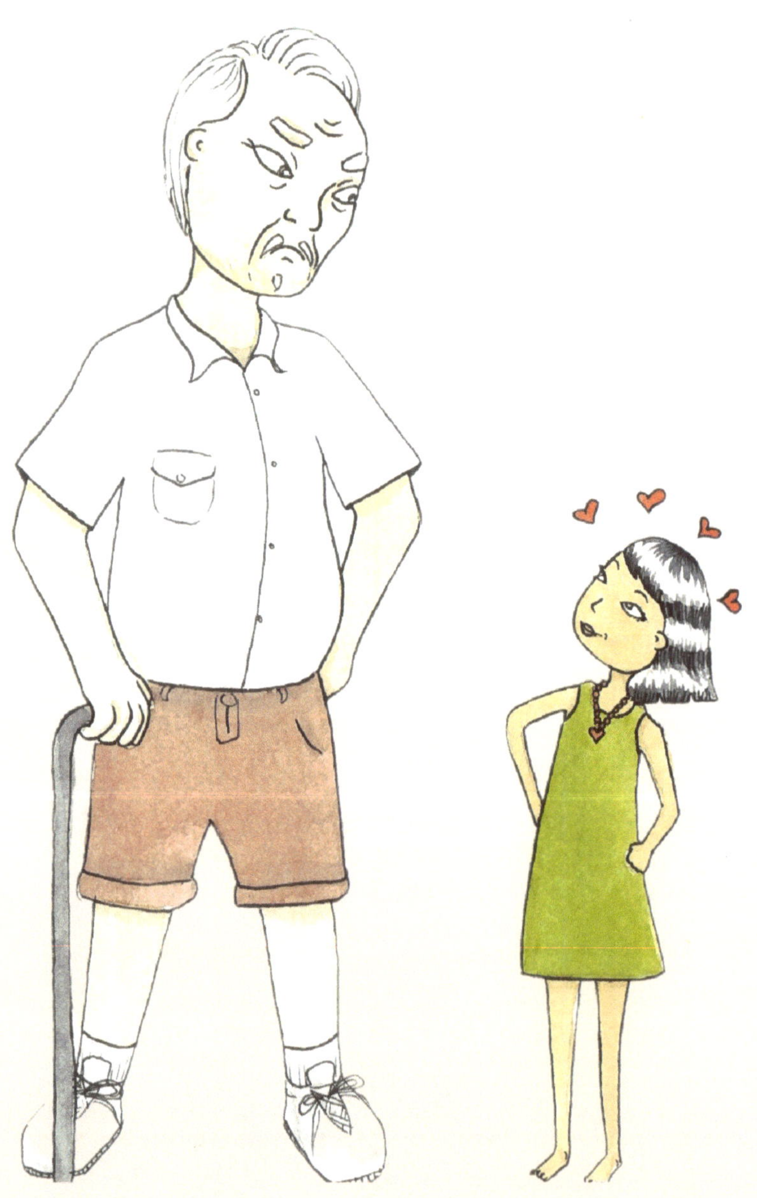

Write down a happy memory you have with your daddy.

Daddy's got **dementia**
But it's **OK**
We can no longer **dance**, but we can **sway**.

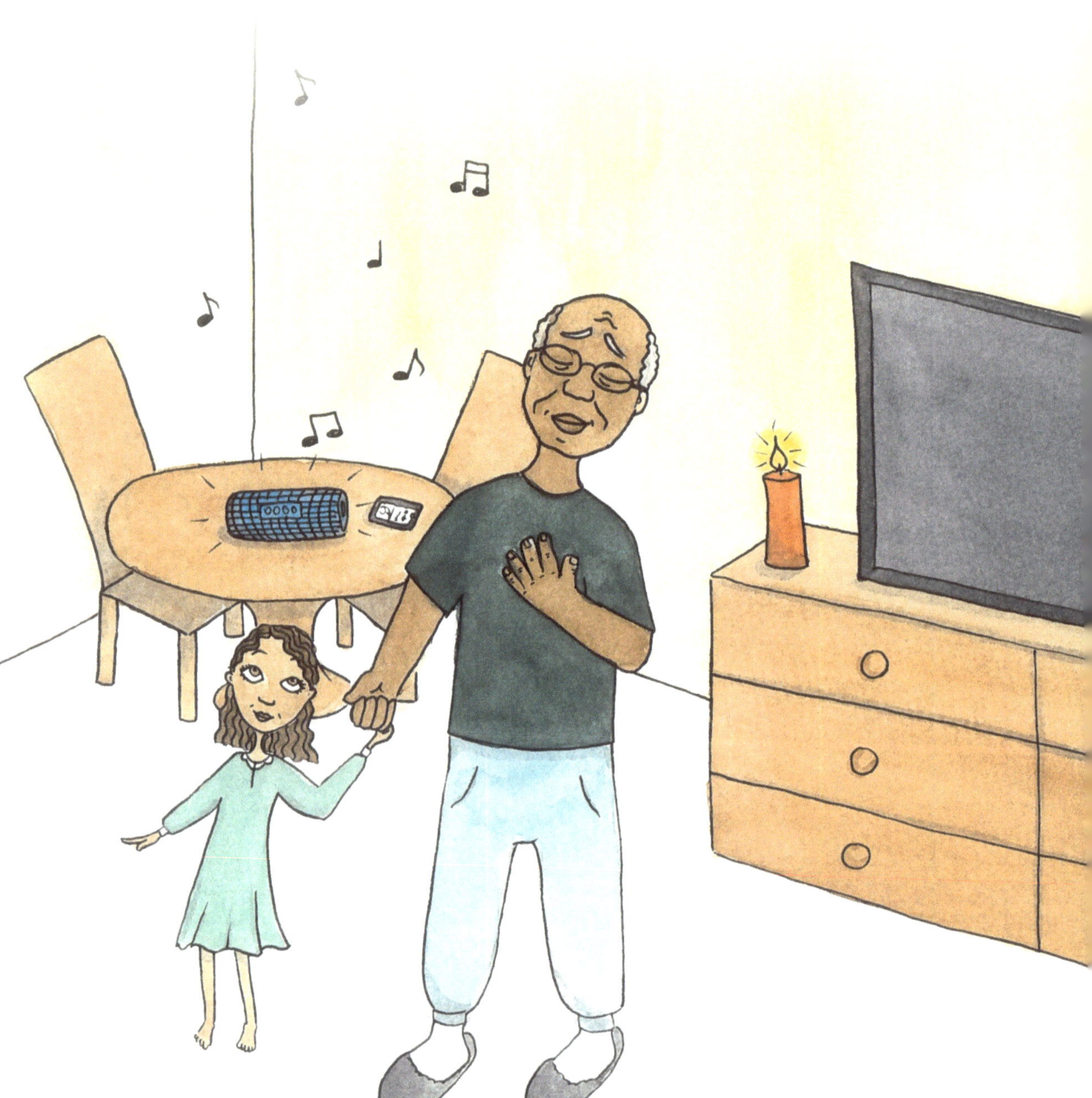

What song reminds you of the good times with your daddy?

Do you have any happy memories that you want to share?

Daddy's got dementia
But it's OK
His nurse is really lovely and she helps him day to day

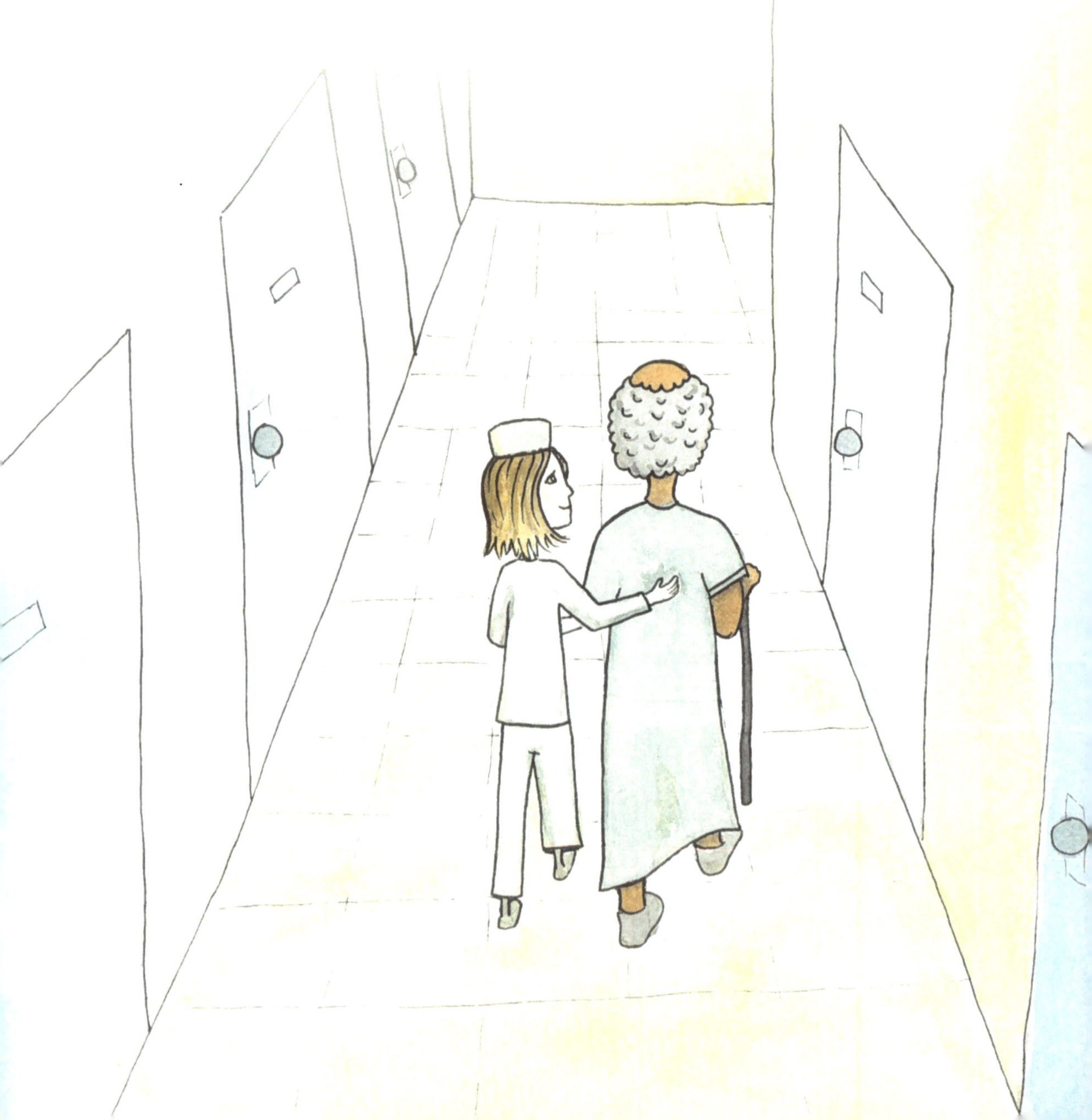

What are your favorite things to do to help daddy?

Daddy's got dementia
But it's OK
We still get to celebrate every holiday

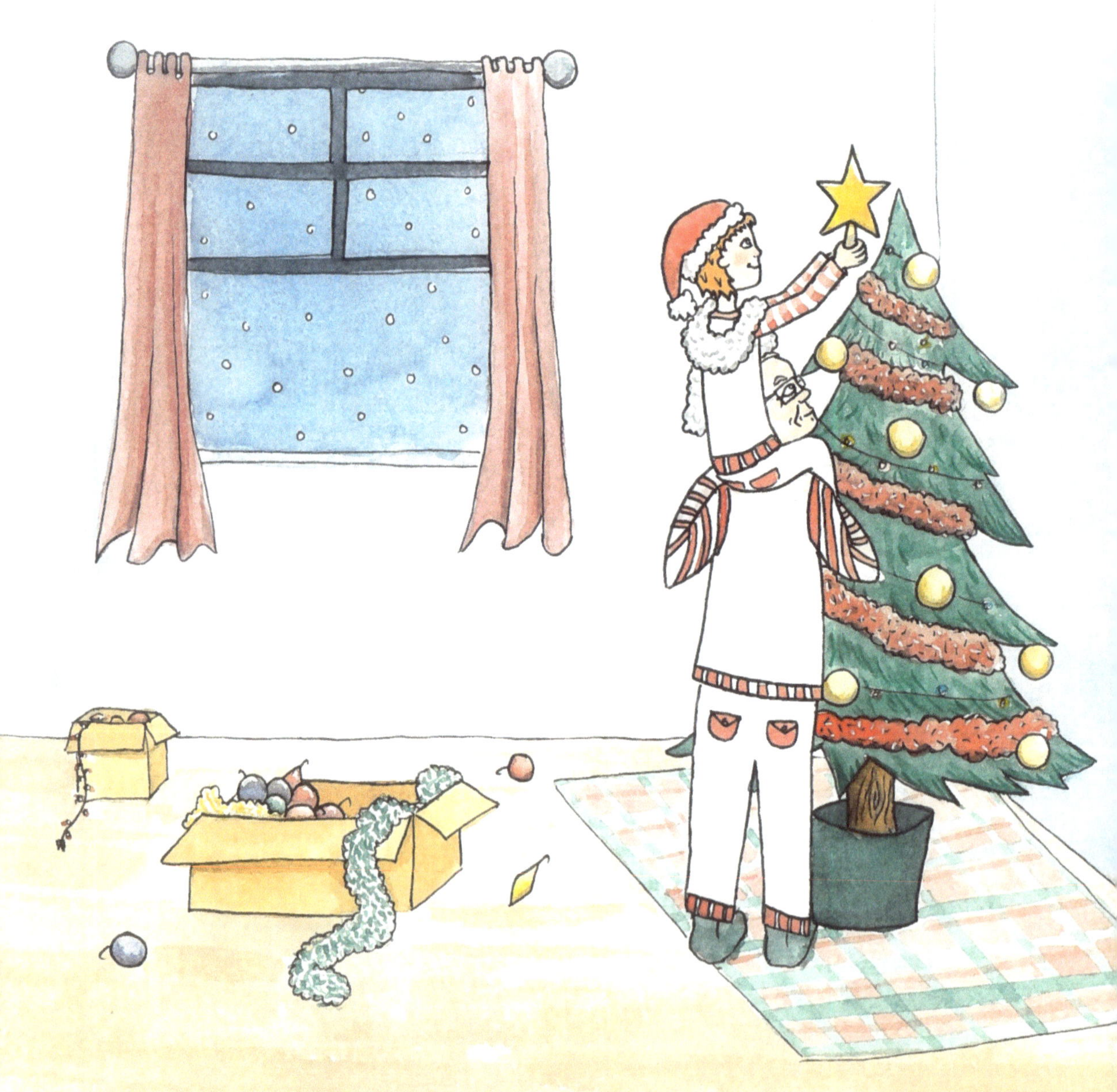

Write down your favorite holiday memory with your daddy?

____

____

____

____

____

____

____

Place a picture of you and daddy at your favorite holiday

Place a picture of you and daddy at your favorite holiday

Daddy's got dementia
But it's OK
He can no longer drive, so we
call mom our valet

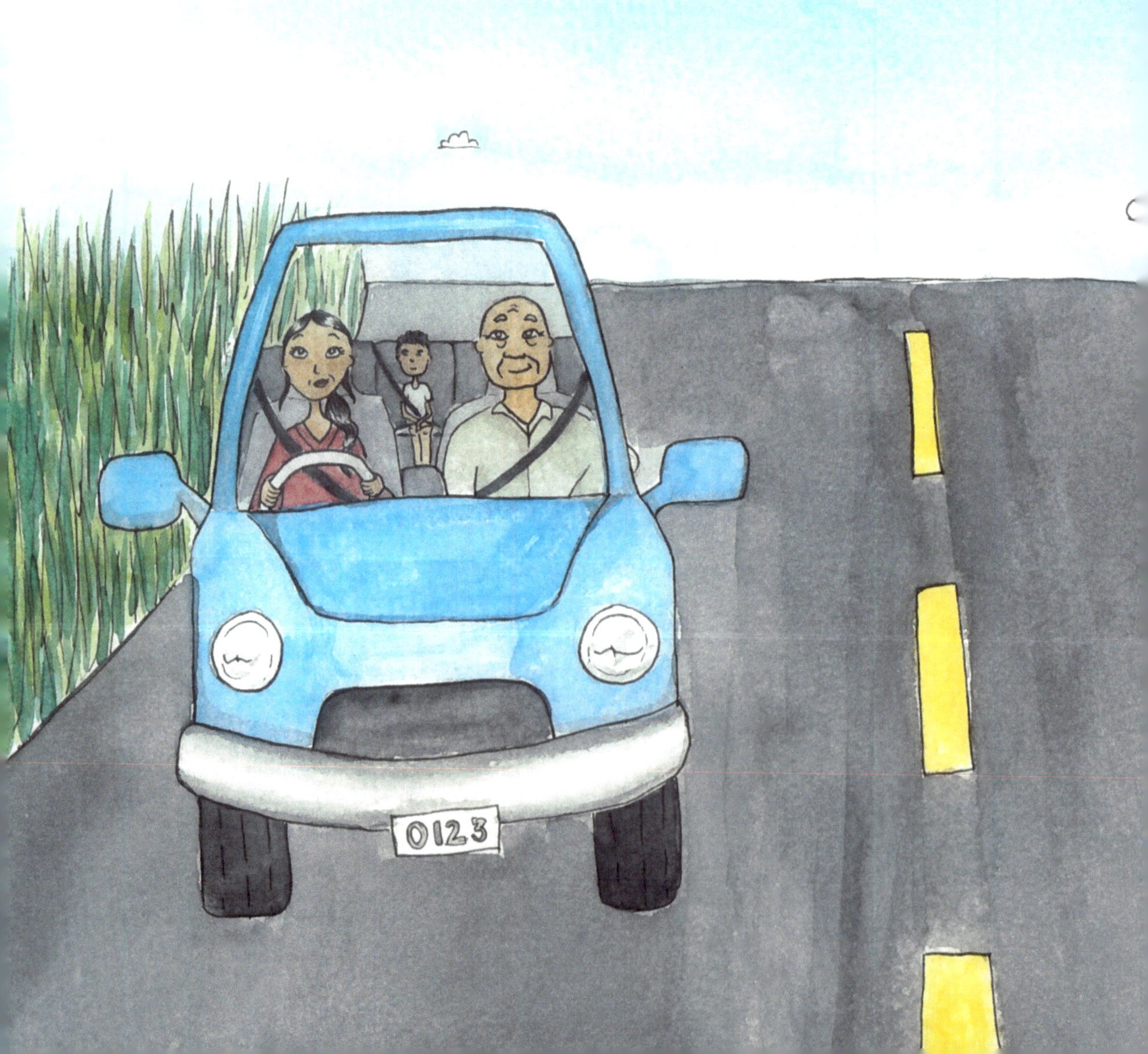

Where is your favorite place to go with your daddy?

Place a happy picture of you and daddy here

Daddy's got **dementia**
But it's **OK**
He made a **mess**, but we **cleaned** it
up **right** away

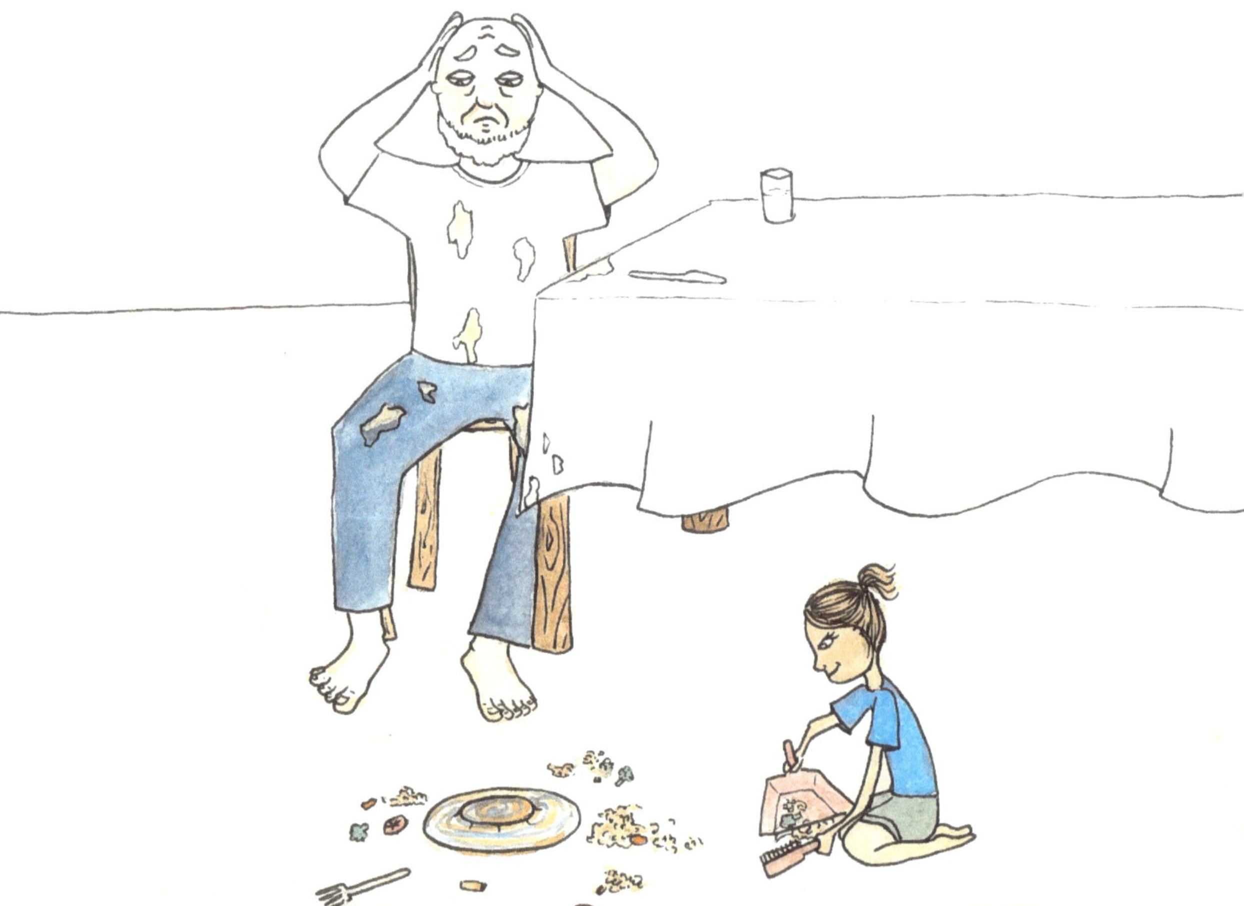

Messes can sometimes be fun, do you have any funny messy memories with your daddy?

Daddy's got **dementia**
But it's **OK**
Even if he's acting **funny** and
things are not the **same**

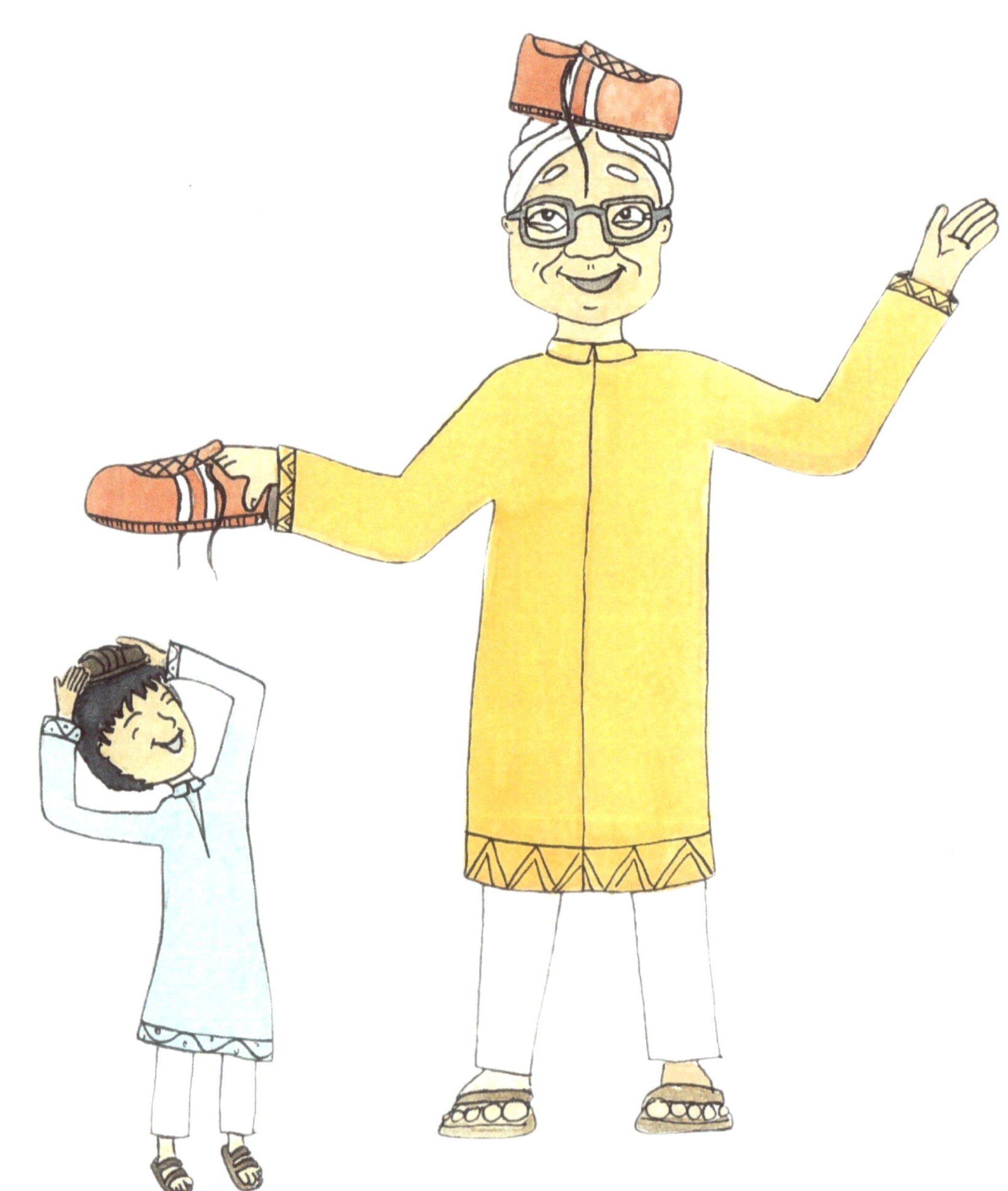

Do you have any funny memories with your daddy?

Daddy's got **dementia**
But it's **OK**
He falls down **sometimes**, so he had to go **away**

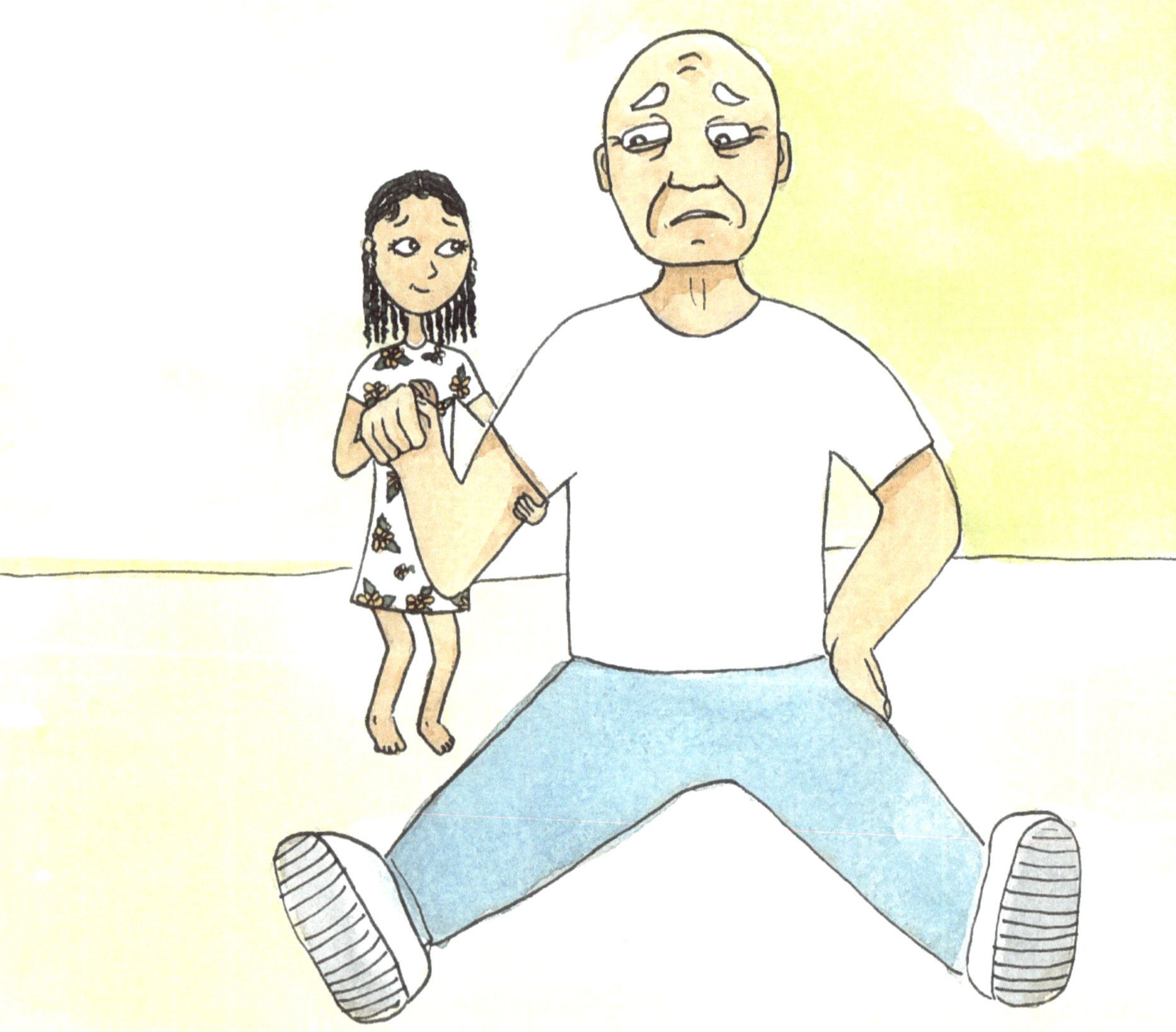

Are there any loving memories about your daddy that may cheer you up?

Daddy's got dementia
But it's OK
We still get to visit him everyday

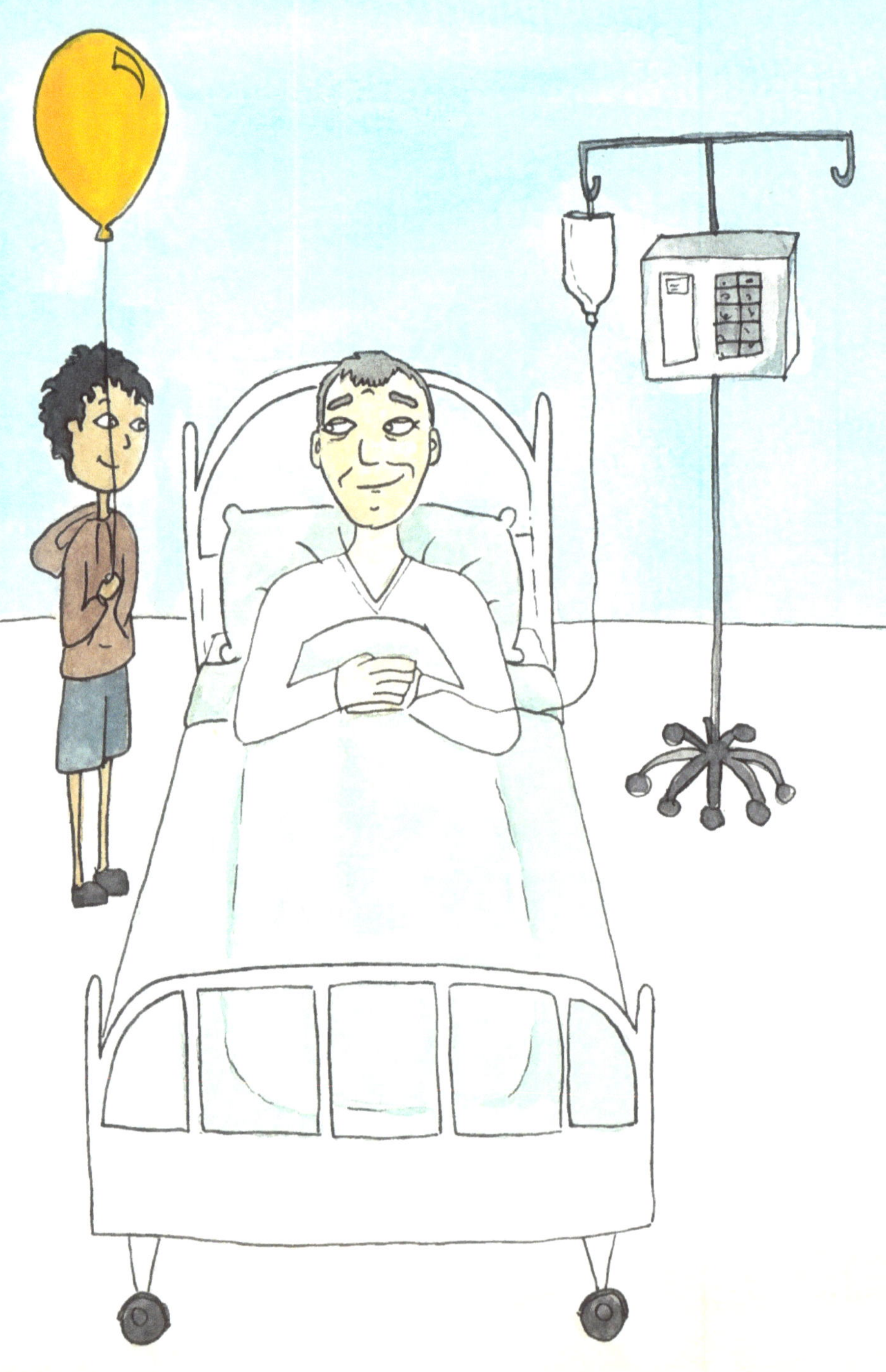

What is a happy memory you have of your daddy?

Place a happy picture of you and daddy here

Daddy's got dementia
But it's OK
We got to visit and bring him
food at his hospital stay.

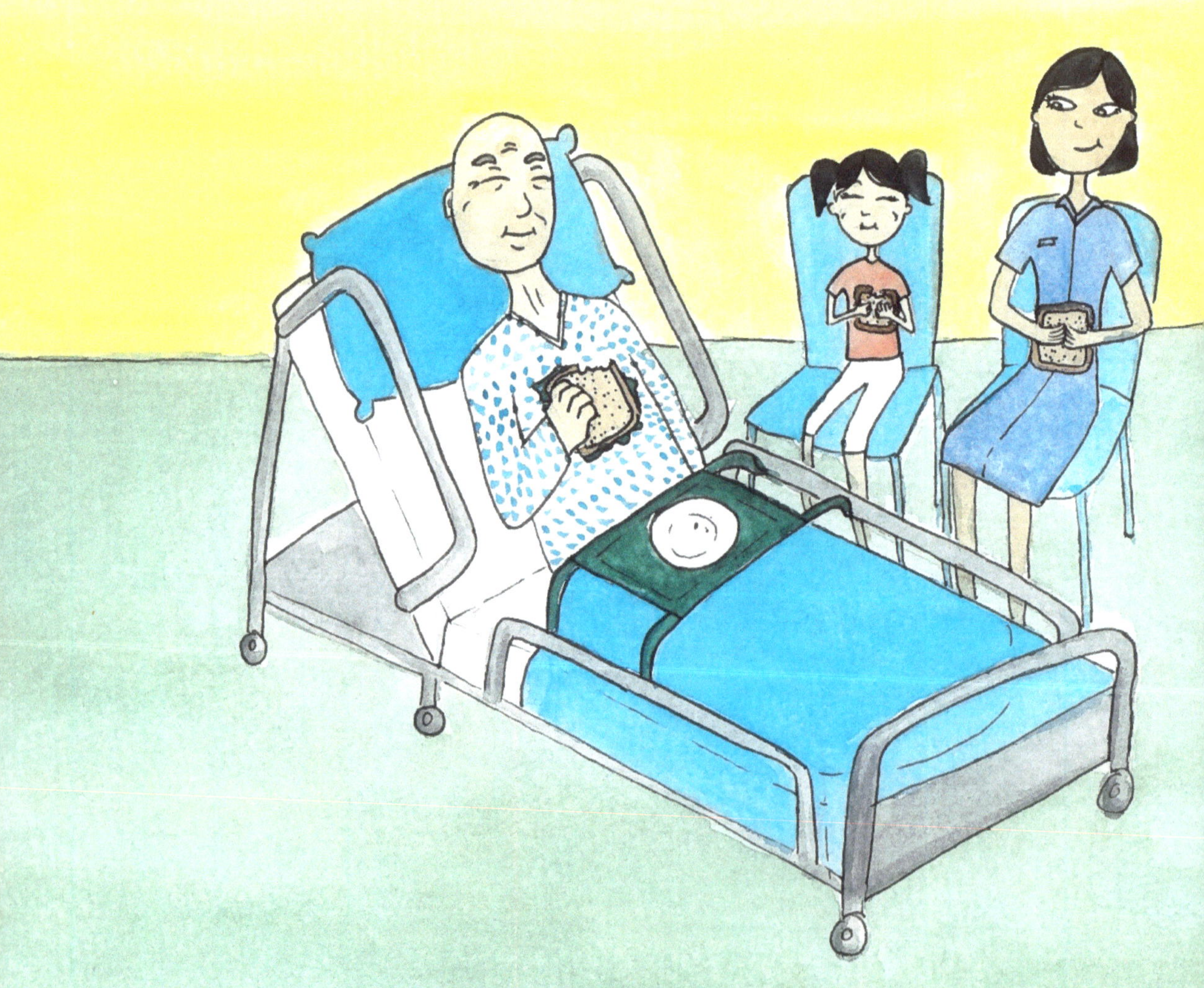

What is daddy's favorite meal/snack in the whole world?

Do you have an interesting story you want to share about your daddy?

Daddy's got dementia
But it's OK
He's not home anymore but he's
still my sunshine ray

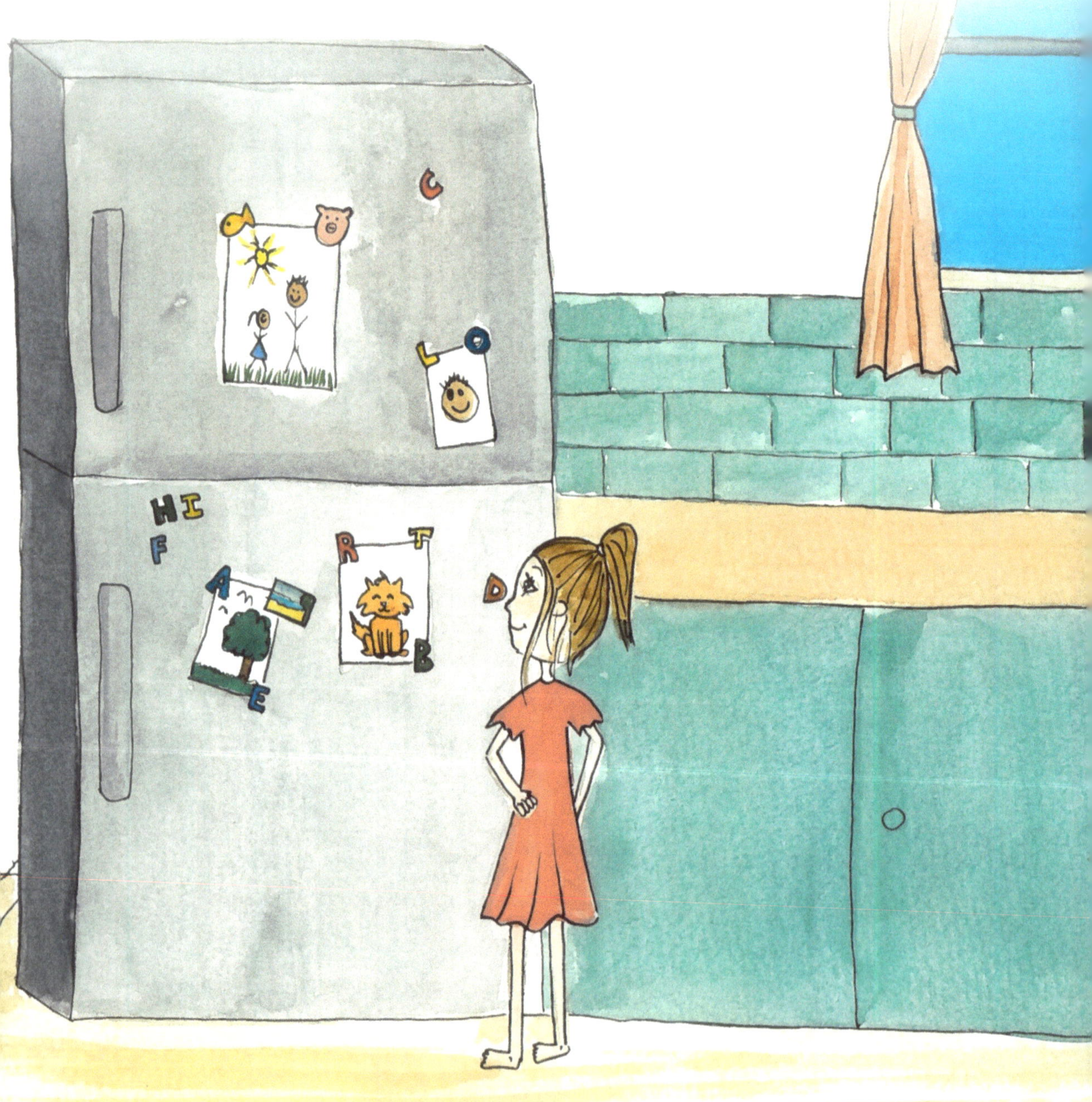

It's OK to miss a loved one, what do you miss the most about your daddy?

Daddy's got dementia
But it's OK
I speak to him every time I pray

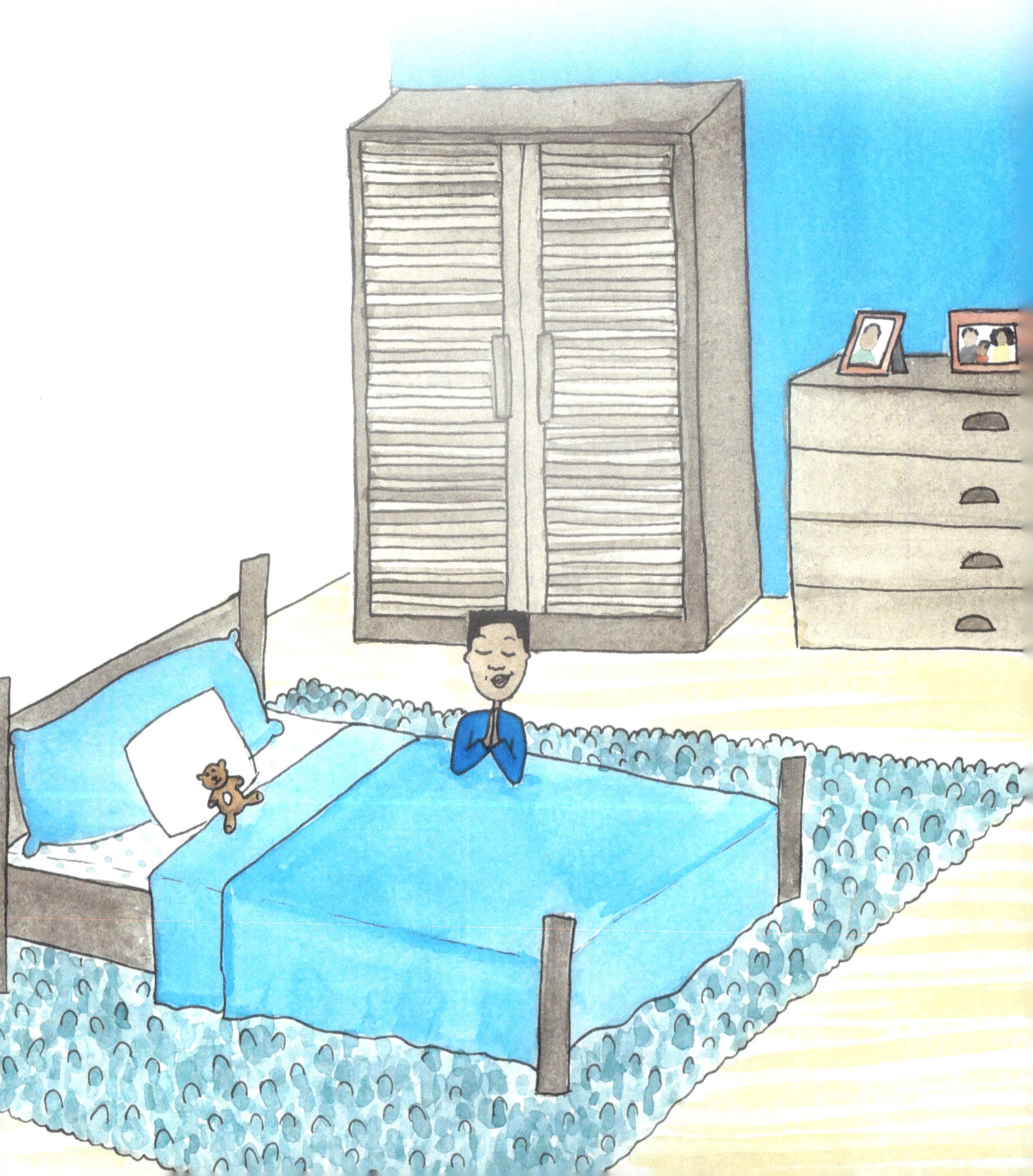

Is there a special memory that you miss about your daddy the most?

Daddy's got dementia
But it's OK
Things may be different now, but our memories are here to stay.

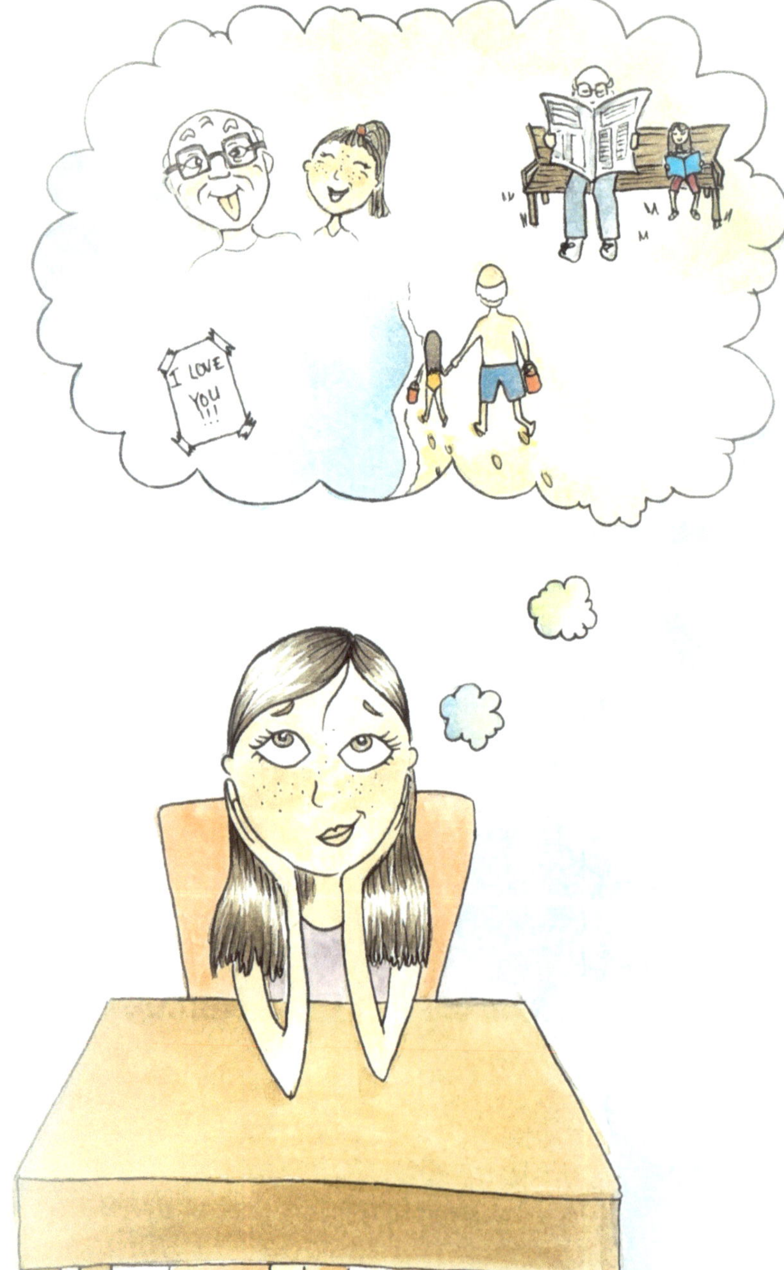

Write down any special memories you want to hold onto forever.

The hardest thing about dementia, is losing someone you love slowly. Here are some questions you can ask so you can remember your loved one forever. And if it ever gets to the point where they are unable to communicate, you can cheer them up with one of their favorite things.

What is daddy's favorite colour?

____

What is daddy's favorite holiday?

____

What is daddy's favorite snack?

____

What is daddy's favorite movie?

____

Can you think of anything else to ask your daddy?

____

____

____

____

____

____

____

____

Dedication

This book is dedicated to my Dad, who I love so much and had the privilege of taking care of throughout his journey with dementia. We had some good times, some funny times and some hard times, but no matter what, we had love, happiness and laughter.

We appreciated every moment, held onto every little memory, and embraced our new journey with open arms.

You were always my biggest cheerleader and I hope to make you proud. Thank you for instilling valuable life lessons, and watching over me, even in sickness you never lost your protective energy. You will be eternally missed, and I wrote this poem for you in honor of our journey together.

Thank you for always having a positive outlook on everything, even during the hardest times, that energy helped me to get through, and made me believe everything would be 'OK.'

You have always been my anchor, but it's time to set sail.
Until we meet again.

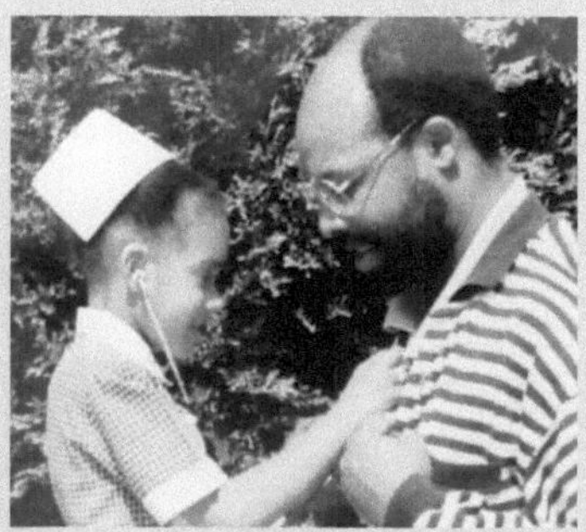